This book belongs to:

_____

(landlady)

And to:

_____

(tenant)

To all the Mama's out there

Pregnancy can be a very challenging time of a woman's life, with all the hormones jumping around your body and a mix of crazy emotions. Every time you feel sad, anxious, crazy, weird, irritated... open this book and read a joke. You will still feel the same, but with a smile on your lips and a warm heart!

I hope this book brings you a little bit of joy and laughter during your pregnancy and that your baby will be a very smiley baby!

Week 1

Success is like pregnancy:
Everybody congratulates you but
nobody knows how many times you
had to get fucked to achieve it.

Week 2

Peeing on a stick and preserving that stick is the start of the many disgusting things you will do as a mother.

Week 3

"I'm proof birth control is 99% effective."

Week 4

How will I know if my vomiting is
morning sickness or the flu?

If it's the flu, you'll get better

Week 5

Prenatal yoga focuses on breathing and stretching. So does napping.

Week 6

"Everybody leave me alone. I've had a busy day being pregnant and I have to do it again tomorrow."

Week 7

A pregnant **woman** has 4 arms, 4 legs, 2 heads, 2 hearts and, possibly, a penis.

Week 8

"Yes, please, whine to me about how tired you are today. Are you growing a human? I didn't think so. Now shut the hell up."

Week 9

"I'm two months pregnant now. When will my baby move?" With any luck, right after he finishes college.

Week 10

How does being pregnant make you feel? "Like a superhero. Well, a really tired, weak superhero who wants to eat all the time and isn't allowed to lift heavy objects."

Week 11

How to win an argument:
(a) Be pregnant.
(b) That's it, you're done!

Week 12

How do you define pregnancy? A nine-month-long hostage situation where you are both the hostage and the building.

Week 13

You don't realize how many people you hate, until you have to name your baby.

Week 14

If you didn't know, you're allowed to eat as much as you want.

"My daily meals include breakfast, lunch, pre-dinner, dinner, pre-dessert, dessert, dessert #2, & a post-dinner snack"

Week 15

"Don't ask me why I am crying
because I don't know."

Week 16

What's the weirdest stage of pregnancy? When people aren't sure whether to congratulate you or hand you some Gas-X.

Week 17

"Since I became pregnant, my breasts, rear-end, and even my feet have grown. Is there anything that gets smaller during pregnancy? Yes, your bladder."

Week 18

Pregnancy is nine months of cheat days.

Week 19

Yelp review for pregnancy:
One out of five stars, took way too long, overpriced, really uncomfortable, too crowded, aesthetically a mess, and no alcohol.

Week 20

5 Stages of Pregnancy:
a) Crying.
b) Peeing.
c) Crying because you peed.
d) Peeing because you're crying.
e) The toilet is your home now.

Week 21

What's better than eating for two while pregnant? Shopping for two.

Week 22

What does a pregnant woman say
after she apologizes for her random
emotional outbursts?
"Up yours and I hate you."

Week 23

"I am pregnant, which means I am sober, swollen, and hungry. Approach with caution."

Week 24

How is a pregnant woman like a toddler? She outgrows her clothes every week!

Week 25

How is being pregnant like being a kid again? There's always someone telling you what to do.

Week 26

A tip for your husband: never, ever
eat the last anything.

Week 27

"If heartburn during pregnancy means you'll have a hairy baby, I'm about to give birth to Chewbacca."

Week 28

"Being pregnant has made me realize it takes talent not to pee yourself when you sneeze."

Week 29

!I am not Buddha. Rubbing my pregnant belly will not bring you good luck."

Week 30

What size pants do you wear?
"Leggings."

Week 31

"Do I have to have a baby shower?"
Not if you change the baby's diaper
very quickly.

Week 32

"Today I told my husband to put the cookies in a place I can't reach... he put them on the floor."

Week 33

Peezing; sneezing and peeing at the same time.

Week 34

Belly rubs: $5.00

Week 35

At 8 months pregnant, one does not simply "roll over in bed".

Week 36

"The only productive part of me today has been my bladder. (Hey, that's something!)"

Week 37

"Yes I'm positive there's just one baby in there. Can I throat punch you now?"

Week 38

Months have an average of 30 days, except the 9th month of pregnancy which has about 1,000 days.

Week 39

"Waiting for this baby is like picking up someone from the airport, but you don't know who they are or what time their flight comes in."

Week 40

Giving Birth is an ecstatic roller coaster ride not available to males.

I hope you had a very good laugh and an amazing pregnancy! Now it's time to open your arms to the most amazing and crazy experience of your entire life! I wish you all the best, don't forget to share with you mama friends (I am sure they will identify themselves too!) and have a great life!

Andie Pi

Printed in Great Britain
by Amazon